BEI GRIN MACHT SICH IHR WISSEN BEZAHLT

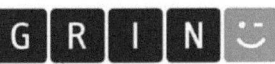

Imprint:

Copyright © 2018 GRIN Verlag
Print and binding: Books on Demand GmbH, Norderstedt Germany
ISBN: 9783668840447

This book at GRIN:

https://www.grin.com/document/450784

Domenic Sommer, Melanie Rossberg, Maria Zander

Driving and Dementia. Assessments to predict the ability to drive

GRIN Verlag

GRIN - Your knowledge has value

Since its foundation in 1998, GRIN has specialized in publishing academic texts by students, college teachers and other academics as e-book and printed book. The website www.grin.com is an ideal platform for presenting term papers, final papers, scientific essays, dissertations and specialist books.

Visit us on the internet:

http://www.grin.com/

http://www.facebook.com/grincom

http://www.twitter.com/grin_com

Driving and Dementia

Assessments to predict the ability to drive

Introduction

▶ Definition: ICD-10-Code F00-F03
  ▷ Not a specific disease → umbrella term that desribes a wide range of symptoms
  ▷ Loss of cognitive functions (thinking, remembering, and reasoning) and behavioral abilities
  ▷ Two core mental funtions must be significantly impaired
    (memory, communication, ability to focus, judgment, visual perception)

▶ Not a natural part of aging (Alzheimer´s association 2018)
  ▷ Dementia isn't always comparable with memory loss issues
  ▷ **BUT:**
    ➢ most patients effeted with the age of 65+
    ➢ Womans having a significant higher risk (Kureckova et al. 2017)

▶ Causes:
  ▷ Nerve cells in the brain stop working, lose connection with other brain cells and die
  ▷ Different types of dementia are associated with particular types of brain cell damage in particular regions of the brain

▶ Different stages and types of dementia

Stages

Early Stage
  ▶ Memory Loss
  ▶ Difficulties with words, time, orientation, places,...
  ▶ Changes in mood & behaviour

Middle Stage
  ▶ Increased memory loss and difficulties with orientation etc.
  ▶ Increased changes in mood & behaviour and inappropriate behavior
  ▶ Issues with personal care and handling complicated tasks

Late Stage
  ▶ Inability to recognize people and items that were familiar
  ▶ No awareness of space and time
  ▶ Issues with mobility, swallowing and possibly incontinence

Types of dementia

- ▶ Alzheimers's Disease
- ▶ Vascular Dementia
- ▶ Dementia with Lewy bodies
- ▶ Mixed Dementia
- ▶ Parkinson's Disease
- ▶ Frantotemporal Dementia
- ▶ Creuzfeldt-Jakob Disease
- ▶ Normals pressure hydrocephalus
- ▶ Huntington's Disease
- ▶ Wernicke-Lorsakoff Syndrome

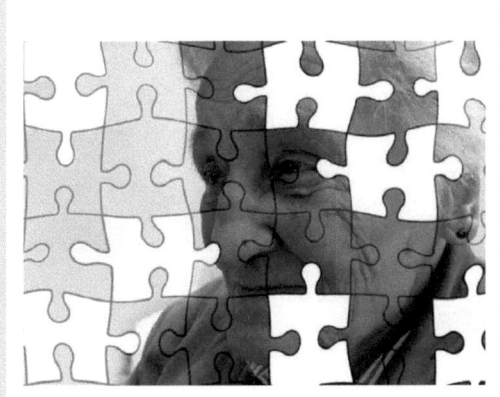

Diagnosis & Therapy

Diagnosis

- ▶ 60% of people with dementia are undiagnosed
- ▶ Diagnosis through
  - ▷ Cognitive and neuropsychological test
    - ▹ Neurological evaluation
    - ▹ Brain scans (CT, MRI, PET scans)
  - ▷ Laboratory tests
  - ▷ Psychiatric evaluation

Therapy

- ▶ Dementia is incurable
- ▶ Therapies is personalized for each dementia patient
- ▶ Medical therapy
- ▶ Non-drug therapy
  - ▷ Biographical approaches
  - ▷ Memory workout
  - ▷ Art therapy
  - ▷ Music therapy
  - ▷ Physiotherapy
  - ▷ Reality orientation training
  - ▷ Pet therapy

Agenda

Driving – A part of life quality

▶ Driving is a part of quality of life
  ▷ Disqualification from driving can cause depression and aggressive behavior
▶ Positive effect:
  ▷ Quality of life, physical and mental health, social interactions trough mobility
▶ Driving is the most important method of transportation
  (Carr et al. 2015)

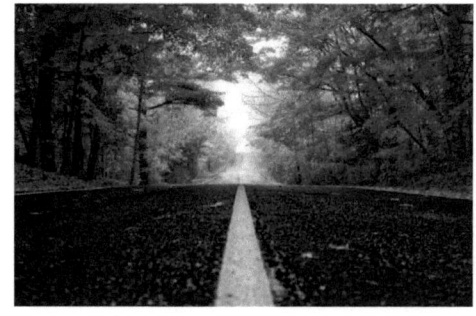

„Driving may be the only way an elder to maintain social contact or provide necessary transportation for self and spouse"
(Dr. Laura B. Brown, PhD, Rhode Island Hospital)

▶ Number of elderly people with a driver license will constantly increase

▶ Number of people with dementia and a driver license will increase as well (Penzek et al. 2015)

▶ **Epidemiology** (Statista GmbH 2017)

▷ Number of patients with dementia worldwide:

▷ **46,8 Mio.**

▷ Number of patients with dementia in Germany:

▷ **1,55 Mio.**

▷ Number of people in Germany driving a car:

▷ **36 Mio.**

▷ **Approximately 658.800 people with dementia have a driver license in Germany**

▷ Demographic change is one of the possible causes for the increasing number of people with dementia

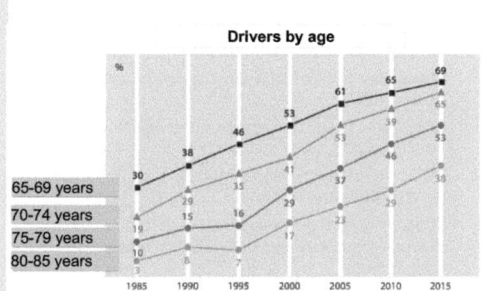

Drivers by age

Display 1:
Significantly more from the older generation:
West Germany, 65- to 85-year-old populations of
1985 to 2015 (Klein et al. 2017, S.109)

▶ **Risk is getting higher with the dementia stages** (Wollny 2008, S.96)

▷ Responsiveness and judgement will be affected (speed, distance,...)

▷ Patients having problems with orientation

▷ Patients driving on the wrong side or take wrong turns

▷ Patients overlooking stop signals and light signals

▶ **Early dementia stage:**
People are having a higher risk but usually they`re able to drive

▶ **Middle to late dementia stage:**
People are mostly unable to drive

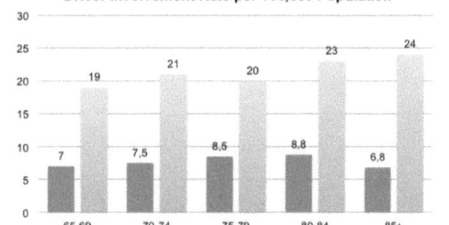

Driver Involvement Rate per 100,000 Population

Display 2:
Involvement Rates for Older Drivers in Fatal Crashes by Age Group and
Gender (NHTSA 2011)

Connection - Driving and Dementia

▶ Evaluation of driving ability

  ▷ The patients doctor should point out the risk of driving with dementia to the patient

  ▷ It's a duty of care but a „grey zone" in most of the countries

  ▷ Germany: regulation of drivers licenses is the duty of the state and not of the doctor

  ▷ Doctors insecurity regarding patients ability to drive a vehicle (Pentzek et al. 2015)

  ▷ Legally secure evaluation of the ability to drive just though a public health officer, traffic medicine department

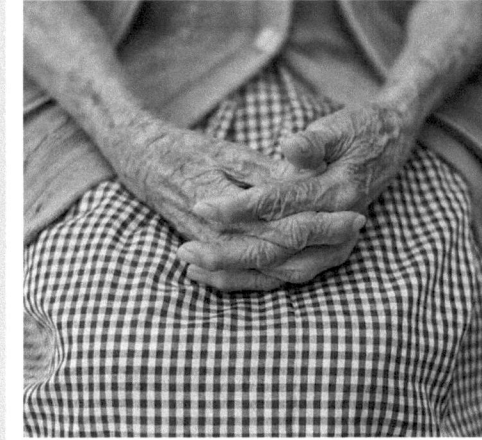

Agenda

▶ **Patient or family report**

▶ **MMSE (Mini-Mental-State Examination)**
  ▷ Most common screening instruments for dementia
  ▷ 30-point (11 questions)

▶ **3MS (Modified Mini-Mental-State Examination)**
  ▷ 3MS is an extended test for MMSE
  ▷ Covering 4 added test items

▶ **AMTS (Abbreviated Mental Test Score)**
  ▷ Used to test for confusion and other cognitive impairments
  ▷ The test consists of 10 questions

▶ **Driving simulation**
  ▷ Safely and efficiently assess and train impaired drivers under hazardous conditions that could never be controlled or tolerated in real world driving (Health Check, Brake reaction test, Knowledge of current road rules)

▶ **RDB (Rookwood Driving Battery)**
  ▷ Content of simple neuropsychological tests (12) designed to assess basic cognitive functions essential for safe driving comprises
  ▷ Visual perception, practical skills and executive function

▶ **DDSA (Dementia Drivers Screening Assessment)**
  ▷ Cognitive test for recommending people with dementia to drive a car
  ▷ This test includes many different neuropsychological test (Stroop Color and Word Test, Visual Object and Space Perception, Road Sign Recognition)

▶ **NADD (Nottingham Assessment for Drivers with Dementia)**
  ▷ Comprises of a series of time limited tasks such as pictorial traffic problems, various written memory tests, speed tests, and visual-perceptual tests

On-Road-Testing

▶ Measures both, the operative maneuvering and cognitive aspects of driving

▶ Assessed with a special observational scoring sheet and a trained driving instructor

▶ 25 road maneuvers, such as turning left and merging with traffic on main roads

▶ Carried out with the participant own car

▶ Driving assessments last approximately 40 minutes

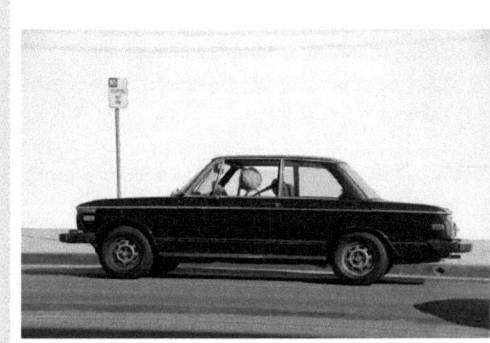

Agenda

Leading Question

▶**Problem:**
There are hardly concrete recommendations regarding dementia and driving.

▶**Question:**
Are cognitive assessments the right way to forecast the driving ability of people with dementia?

▶**Destination:**
Our main goal was to derive an overall recommendation which test should be used
and furthermore to identify research demands.

Agenda

1   Dementia - A short introduction

2   Driving - Relevance of the topic

3   Assessments

4   Focus

5   Methodology

6   Results

7   Discussion

8   Conclusion & Recommendation

9   References

Methodology

- ▶ Systematic research in PubMed and EBSCO
- ▶ Synonyms and MeshTerms were used for different words
- ▶ Search terms were used individually and in combination
- ▶ Selection of search terms:
  dementia, Alzheimer*, driving, automobile, motor, vehicle, off-road-assessments, cognitive measurements, neuropsych*, mini mental state examination
- ▶ Incremental hand search in Gerontological Society of America
- ▶ Only articles in english were chosen
- ▶ Studies were first filtered trough Abstract und Title
- ▶ 6 studies were downloaded and read completely
- ▶ Quality of the assessments:
  - ▷ Quantitative Studies via CONSORT Checklist (Version 2010)
  - ▷ Systematic Reviews via AMSTAR

Search strategy

Tab. 1: search strategy in data bases

#	Search terms	EBSCO (n)	PubMed (n)
1	operate a car OR driving OR driver OR motor vehicle OR automobile OR traffic	1.692.256	179.096
2	dementia or alzheimers or cognitive impairment or memory loss) OR dementia patients OR cognitive deficits	171.803	301.187
3	1 and 2	1.891	2.827
4	psychological gerontology OR off-road assessments OR cognitive measures OR neuropsychological assessment OR neuropsychological measures OR mmse or mini mental state examination	34.032	207.546
5	3 and 4	153	666
6	Filter: published date → 2012 - 2018	85	234
7	5 NOT driving behavior NOT pedestrian NOT walking NOT crossing NOT sleep NOT nighttime driving NOT alcohol NOT sedation medication NOT opiod NOT medication NOT pain killers	67	155
8	7 and ((randomized controlled trials or rtc or randomised control trials) OR random OR placebo OR controlled clinical trial OR cct OR systematic review OR review OR (meta-analysis or systematic review or literature review or meta analysis or overview) OR (guidlines or recommendation))	9	33

Selection of Studies

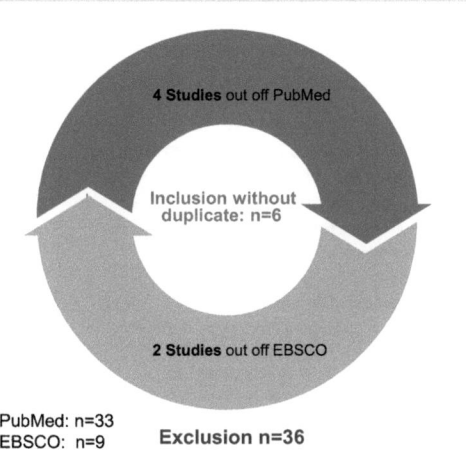

PubMed: n=33
EBSCO: n=9   **Exclusion n=36**

Exclusion criteria:
- ▶ Multimorbidity than other diseases as dementia
- ▶ Assessments not part of study design
- ▶ Other Tests (driving simulator, on-road-tests)
- ▶ Pedestrians
- ▶ Microsleep and nighttime driving
- ▶ Driving under the influence of drugs, alcohol and medicines (pain killers, sedation medicine,...)

Inclusion criteria:
- ▶ Evaluation of the forecasting power of cognitive tests regarding driving with dementia
- ▶ Trustworthy studies with a high evidence level
- ▶ Randomized studies
- ▶ Systematic reviews

Agenda

1   **Dementia - A short introduction**

2   **Driving - Relevance of the topic**

3   **Assessments**

4   **Focus**

5   **Methodology**

6   Results

7   **Discussion**

8   **Conclusion & Recommendation**

9   **References**

Results
Study by Seiler et al. 2012:
"Driving cessation and dementia results of the prospective registry on dementia in Austria"

Characteristic

- ▶ Cohort study with a high variation of cognitive tests **but** no randomisation
- ▶ Mean age: 74,2 years
- ▶ Assessments: MMSE, CERAD, CDR, ADL (disability assessment for dementia)
- ▶ n = 240 dementia cases who were car-drivers (from Austria)
- ▶ Multivarite analysis (logistic regression)
- ▶ Publisher: PRODEM Study Group, medical university of graz, Austria

Study outcome

- ▶ Gender has a significant part when it comes to disqualification from driving by choice
- ▶ Highest Rate of driving cessation in the study population
  - ▷ 90,9% with lewy body dementia (LBD)
  - ▷ 58,2% with alzheimers disease (AD)
- ▶ Reasons for driving cessation:
  - ▷ High risk reported mostly by their caregivers
  - ▷ Self-responsibility in people with dementia
- ▷ Safety of driving with dementia
  - ▷ Low Rate of accidents (8 of 240)
  - ▷ People disqualified from driving mostly effected by a higher MMSE/CERAD (disabilities, late dementia stage)
- ▶ Significant factor of driving cessation:
  - ▷ Demography, female gender, constructional abilities on CERAD and impairment in activity of daily life (ADL)

Results
Study by Vella and Lincoln 2014:
„Comparison of assessment of fitness to drive for people with dementia in UK"

Characteristic

- ▶ Study with a small group of participants in the UK
- ▶ Mean age were 74,1 years
- ▶ 18man/6 females
- ▶ 24 patients were recruited by mental health teams and psychiatrist
- ▶ Two batteries were used (Rockwood Driving Battery (RDB) & Dementia Drivers Screening Assessment (DDSA))
- ▶ Each participant were assessed on both tests
- ▶ Publisher: Institute of Work, Health and Organizations, University of Nottingham (UK)

Study outcome

- ▶ Neuropsychological batteries designed to assist to inform recommendations about the fitness to drive
  - ▷ Rockwood Driving Battery (RDB)
  - ▷ Dementia Drivers´Screening Assessment (DDSA)
- ▶ Comparing any discordant classifications against on-road driving ability with the passing or failing of the RDB or DDSA
- ▶ Those with discrepant results had to do an on-road test as well
- ▶ Potential participants needed to have an diagnosis with dementia, needed to speak english, without any other medical diagnosis that could affect their performance on the cognitive batteries, had driven vehicle within the last two years, ...
- ▶ On-road testing were conducted using the participants own cars
- ▶ Problem: RDB is classifying individuals as unsafe to drive, who are classified as safe by the DDSA
- ▶ Most participants with dementia were found to be unsafe to drive
- ▶ Highly positive predictive value, so that those who fail the RDB are likely to be unsafe drivers
- ▶ RDB is stricter than the DDSA , DDSA is better at identifying safe drivers than unsafe driver

esults
tudy by Carr and O'Neil 2015:
Mobility and safety issues in drivers with dementia"

Characteristic

- Literature review who evaluates assessments of dementia severity in relation to driving
- Mean age: 75 years
- Systematic Review: wasn't recognizable in the search
- High spectrum of themes
  - Assessments, role and point of view of the doctors
- Different outcomes:
  - Safety, driving related deaths/injuries, Driving Cessation etc.
- Publisher: Washington University (St. Louis), Trinity Centre for Health Sciences (Ireland)

Study outcome

- Driving outcomes (crash risk, driving performance by on-road tests)
  - differ between dementia severity (Clinical Dementia Rating)
  - differ between types of dementia (lewy body dementia und alzheimer disease = more deficits)
- Safety in early dementia stages is comparable to drivers without dementia
- MMSE correlates with degree of driving impairment on road tests
  - The MMSE scores can provide a rough estimate of dementia severity and possibly driving risk
  - Psychometric tests should:
    - be used together with other tests
    - include the risk by medication and comorbidities
    - include the evaluation of family members or caregivers
- Benefits of driving evaluations should consider a closer look

esults
tudy by Martin et al. 2013:
Driving for maintaining mobility and safety in drivers with dementia"

Characteristic

- Systematic intervention review
- Association between cognitive measures and driver safety
- 63 full text papers reviewed plus 2nd search with 70 abstract screening
- No study reviewed has discussed long-term transport mobility outcomes for people who passed of failed evaluations
- On-road testing as gold standard
- Further research is needed regarding neuropsychological tests
- Publisher: The Cochrane Collaboration and published in the Cochrane Library

Study outcome

- No benefit of driving assessments has yet been prospectively demonstrated
  - No evidence that driving assessment helps to maintain mobility or improve safety for drivers with dementia
  - Indicates the need of more research and need of standardized diver assessment models (for dementia)
  - Screening appears to discriminate against older drivers
- Driving simulators aren't the right comparison with cognitive assessments
- Driving simulators are not comparable with an on-road test
  - Control group in this study is critical
- Different dementia types: Differences of the Assessment/ Driving Performance
  - Alzheimers disease is the most iresearched type of dementia and has the highest effect of the fitness to drive

Study by Bennett et al. 2016:
"Cognitive Test and Determining Fitness to Drive in Dementia"

Characteristic

- Systematic Review
- Investigates the relationship between cognitive assessment and driving performance of individuals with dementia
- Selection of studies include initial screen of title and abstract (260 articles)
- 35 studies were reviewed in full text
- Used Assessment:
  - Newcastle-Ottawa Quality Assessment Scale for Cohort and Case Control Studies
- Publisher: Macquarie University Sydney

Study outcome

- Results of individual tests were variable
  - MMSE most commonly used individual test with 14 of the 25 findings (56%) - showed positive association with driving
- TMT-A and TMT-B important tests
  - 6 times with positive association
  - TMT-B 8 times with 3 showings of positive association
  - Single tests should not be used as indicators of fitness to drive because they are not sufficient to obtain a reliable picture of driving ability
- Test batteries:
  - Results are indifferent
  - One author has a positive association and the other author has none
  - Relevance of other tests:
    - cognitive domain, visuospatial skills, memory, attention progressing speed, language seem to be more important to assess driving outcomes

---

Study by Smedslund et al. 2015:
"Screening tools for cognitive function and driving"

Characteristic

- Systematic review
- About the accuracy of cognitive screening tests designed to predict results on standardized driving tests
- 53 studies fulfilled the inclusion criteria
  - exclusively off-road-tests
- Has a control group
  - simulator as reference, on road test
- Large variation of off-roads tests (MMSE, Montreal Cognitive Assessment, Clock Drawing Test, Trail Making Test-B, etc.)
- Publisher: Norwegian Knowledge Center for the Health Services, Haukeland University Hospital

Study outcome

- Didn't find any studies with accidents as outcome
- There was a large variability between the studies both for sensitivity and specificity
- They didn´t find cognitive screening test that have high quality evidence for diagnostic test accuracy for predicting driving ability assessed with on-road test
- Test with the most significance:
  - Montreal Cognitive Assessment 70-85% (sensitivity)
  - Clock Drawing Test 65-71%,
  - Trail-Making Test B 70-77%

Quality of included studies: AMSTAR

Question	Systematic Review			Literature reviews (systematic not clear)
	Martin et. al.	Bennett et. al.	Smegdslund et. al.	Carr et. al.
1. Was an 'a priori' design provided?	Yes	Not clear	Yes	No
2. Was there duplicate study selection and data extraction?	Yes	No	Yes	No
3. Was a comprehensive literature search performed?	Yes	Yes	Yes	Not clear
4. Was a comprehensive literature search performed?	No	No	Yes	Not clear
5. Was a list of studies (included and excluded) provided?	Yes	Yes	Yes	Yes
6. Were the characteristics of the included studies provided?	Not applicable	Yes	Yes	No

Quality of included studies: AMSTAR

Question	Systematic Reviews			Literature reviews (systematic not clear)
	Martin et. al.	Bennett et. al.	Smegdslund et. al.	Carr et. al.
7. Was the scientific quality of the included studies assessed and documented?	Not applicable	Yes	Yes	Yes
8. Was the scientific quality of the included studies used appropriately in formulating conclusions?	Not applicable	Yes	Yes	No
9. Were the methods used to combine the findings of studies appropriate?	Not applicable	Yes	Yes	Yes
10. Was the likelihood of publication bias assessed?	Not applicable	Yes	Yes	No
11. Was the conflict of interest included?	No	Yes	No	Yes

Quality of included studies: CONSORT

CONSORT-Elements	Seiler et al. 2012	Vella et al.
Title and Summary	2 (2)	0,5 (2)
Introduction and background	1,5 (2)	1,5 (2)
Methods		
Trial design	2 (2)	1,5 (2)
Participants	2 (2)	2 (2)
Interventions/ Treatments	1 (1)	0,5 (1)
Outcomes	1,5 (2)	0,5 (2)
Sample size	0,5 (2)	0,5 (2)
Randomisation		
Sequence generation	0 (2)	0,5 (2)
Allocation concealment mechanism	0 (1)	0,5 (1)
Implementation	0 (1)	0,5 (1)
Blinding	0,5 (2)	1,5 (2)
Statistical methods	2 (2)	0,5 (2)

Quality of included studies: CONSORT

CONSORT-Elements	Seiler et al. 2012	Vella et al.
Results		
In- and exclusion criteria	2 (2)	0,5 (2)
Recruitment	2 (2)	0 (2)
Patient characteristica (baseline data)	1 (1)	0,5 (1)
Numbers analysed	1 (1)	1 (1)
Outcomes and stimation	1,5 (2)	0,5 (2)
Chats/ Illustration	0,5 (1)	0,5 (1)
Additional analysis	0 (1)	0 (1)
Harms	0 (1)	0 (1)
Discussion		
Limitiations	1 (1)	1 (1)
Generalisability	0,5 (1)	1 (1)
Interpretation	1 (1)	1 (1)
Other Informations		
Registration	0 (1)	0 (1)
Protocol	0 (1)	0 (1)
Funding	1 (1)	0 (1)

scussion
Methodology discussion

▶ **Data collection and analysis**
- ▷ Search strategy (limitation of two databases)
  - ⚞ Could've used more databases
- ▷ Different dementia stages
  - ⚞ Could've used a specialization like Alzheimers
- ▷ No specialization of a group of age
- ▷ Focus on dementia in general

▶ **Data extraction**
- ▷ Several authors reviewed all studies independently from each other
- ▷ No checklist used for results
- ▷ Tried to use a consistent demonstration
- ▷ Filtered for the same criteria

▶ **Quality Assessment**
- ▷ Several authors reviewed all studies independently from each other
- ▷ Discussion afterwards

Outcome discussion

- ▶ Practicability questionable for Germany
  - ▷ Located evidence referred to different countries
  - ▷ A lot of differences in all the countries at handling the ability of the fitness to drive

- ▶ Driving cessation leads to conflict of interest
  - ▷ Automotive industry would sell less cars
  - ▷ Elderly people are spending more money for new vehicles
  - ▷ Probably reason for low number of studies

- ▶ Assessments are building risks:
  - ▷ Drivers that don't pass the assessments may be:
    - ≻ a the risk to shift to more dangerous modes of transportation
    - ≻ more vulnerable in traffic in general

- ▶ People with dementia ar getting enough help from society
- ▶ Society disadvantages elderly people in general, even more if they're confused

Outcome discussion

- ▶ It seems, that other factors are more important
  - ▷ Other assessments
    - ≻ Tests of the eye vision
    - ≻ Diagnostic of comorbidities (especially heart disease instead of dementia)
  - ▷ Caregivers und families are important for the decision making progress when it comes to handing out driver's license
  - ▷ Gender: womans are more likely to cease driving than men
- ▶ Single tests, like the MMSE, are not designed to determine indicators of fitness to drive
  - ▷ But they are usually used by physicians, caregivers, etc. (Bennet et al. 2016, S. 1915)
  - ▷ Not enough evidence about the effectiveness of driving assessments:
    - ≻ Lack of standardized outcome measures
    - ≻ Low study population, no significance
    - ≻ Outcome factors of driving with dementia are difficult to measure
    - ≻ No results for the ultimate outcomes: traffic accidents
- **BUT:**
  - ▷ In general: matches with Canadian Consensus Conference of dementia and older reviews

Outcome discussion

▶ Decision of driving cessation should not be taken lightly
  ▷ Driving cessation has been associated with:
    ➢ Decrease in social integration
    ➢ Decreased out-of-home-activities
    ➢ Increase in depressive and anxiety symptoms
    ➢ Increased risk of nursing home placement…

▶ Driving-Alternatives must be considered:
  ▷ Not enough help from society
  ▷ To few transport services for people with dementia
  ▷ Higher expenses through taxi vouchers, bus tickets, …

▶ Mobility counselling gets more important (Carr and O'Neill 2015)
  ▷ Patients need alternatives to driving
  ▷ Further education for doctors for dementia assessments
  ▷ Option to consult with an mobility expert as a prevention method

Agenda

1 Dementia - A short introduction

2 Driving - Relevance of the topic

3 Assessments

4 Focus

5 Methodology

6 Results

7 Discussion

8 Conclusion & Recommendation

9 References

Conclusion

- ▶ Dementia awareness is still too low
- ▶ Single tests insufficient
- ▶ General Assumption: To many drivers with dementia
- ▶ Issue should be more sensitized
- ▶ No clear evidence regarding the assessment
- ▶ Not enough literature and information

- ▶ **BEST CASE:** Combination of off- and on-road test (battery tests)
  - ▷ Suitable for predicting fitness to drive in dementia
    - ⊁ RDB (Rookwood Driving Battery)
    - ⊁ DDSA (Dementia Drivers Screening Assessment)
    - ⊁ NADD (Nottingham Assessment for Drivers with dementia)

Recommendation

▶ Do's

- ▷ More standardization in the outcome measures
- ▷ More research needed in psychometric tests and driving performance
- ▷ Frequent medical evaluation of the ability to drive in high-risk groups (dementia, heart disease, etc.)
- ▷ Doctor as a lawyer of the patient:
  - ▷ A doctor should:
    - ⊁ give advice on driving ability
    - ⊁ decide carefully
    - ⊁ use the relationship with the patient

▶ Don'ts:

- ▷ Discrimination against vulnerable groups (elderly patients with dementia)
- ▷ Limitation for driving of elderly people
  - ▷ No disadvantage of elderly people in country areas
- ▷ No stigmatization

Agenda

References

Alzheimer´s association (Hg.) (2018): Alzheimer's Disease. Online verfügbar unter https://alz.org/alzheimers_disease_1973.asp, zuletzt aktualisiert am 12.01.2018, zuletzt geprüft am 13.01.2018.

Bennett, Joanne M.; Chekaluk, Eugene; Batchelor, Jennifer (2016): Cognitive Tests and Determining Fitness to Drive in Dementia. A Systematic Review. In: *Journal of the American Geriatrics Society* 64 (9), S. 1904–1917. DOI: 10.1111/jgs.14180.

Brown, Laura B.; Ott, Brian R. (2004): Driving and dementia. A review of the literature. In: *Journal of geriatric psychiatry and neurology* 17 (4), S. 232–240. DOI: 10.1177/0891988704269825.

Carr, David B.; O'Neill, Desmond (2015): Mobility and safety issues in drivers with dementia. In: *International psychogeriatrics* 27 (10), S. 1613–1622. DOI: 10.1017/S104161021500085X.

Generali Deutschland AG (Hg.) (2017): Generali Altersstudie 2017. Berlin, Heidelberg: Springer Berlin Heidelberg.

Klein, Thomas; Rapp, Ingmar (2017): Alltag und digital Medien. In: Generali Deutschland AG (Hg.): Generali Altersstudie 2017. Berlin, Heidelberg: Springer Berlin Heidelberg, S. 89–119.

Kurečková, V.; Trepáčová, M.; Zaoral, A.; Řezáč, P.; Zámečník P. (2017): Should patients with dementia be allowed to drive. In: *Geriatrie a Gerontologie* 6 (54), S. 126–129.

Martin, Alan J.; Marottoli, Rrichard; O'Neill, Desmond (2013): Driving assessment for maintaining mobility and safety indrivers with dementia (Review). In: *Cochrane Database of Systematic Reviews* 5 (CD006222), S. 1–35, zuletzt geprüft am 08.01.2018.

Moher, David; Hopewell, Sally; Schulz, Kenneth F.; Montori, Victor; Gøtzsche, Peter C.; Devereaux, P. J. et al. (2010): CONSORT 2010 explanation and elaboration. Updated guidelines for reporting parallel group randomised trials. In: *BMJ (Clinical research ed.)* 340, 1-28. DOI: 10.1136/bmj.c869.

References

Pentzek, Michael; Michel, Jacqueline Verena; Ufert, Marie; Vollmar, Horst Christian; Wilm, Stefan; Leve, Verena (2015): Fahrtauglichkeit bei Demenz - Theoretische Rahmung und Konzept einer Vorgehensempfehlung für die Hausarztpraxis. In: *Zeitschrift fur Evidenz, Fortbildung und Qualitat im Gesundheitswesen* 109 (2), S. 115–123. DOI: 10.1016/j.zefq.2015.03.005.

Seiler, Stephan; Schmidt, Helena; Lechner, Anita; Benke, Thomas; Sanin, Guenter; Ransmayr, Gerhard et al. (2012): Driving cessation and dementia. Results of the prospective registry on dementia in Austria (PRODEM). In: *PloS one* 7 (12), 52-58. DOI: 10.1371/journal.pone.0052710.

Shea, Beverley J.; Grimshaw, Jeremy M.; Wells, George A.; Boers, Maarten; Andersson, Neil; Hamel, Candyce et al. (2007): Development of AMSTAR. A measurement tool to assess the methodological quality of systematic reviews. In: *BMC medical research methodology* 7, S. 10. DOI: 10.1186/1471-2288-7-10.

Smedslund, Geir; Giske, Liv; Fleitscher, Hilde; Brurberg, Kjetil (2015): Screening tools for cognitive function and driving. Report from Norwegian Knowledge Centre for the Health Services (21), zuletzt geprüft am 08.01.2018.

Statista GmbH (Hg.) (2017): Dossier. Autofahrer. Online verfügbar unter https://de.statista.com/statistik/studie/id/7059/dokument/autofahrer-statista-dossier/, zuletzt geprüft am 08.01.2018.

Statista GmbH (Hg.) (2018): Dossier. Demenzerkrankungen. Online verfügbar unter https://de.statista.com/statistik/studie/id/17631/dokument/demenzerkrankungen-statista-dossier/, zuletzt geprüft am 08.01.2018.

Vella, Kristina; Lincoln, Nadina B. (2014): Comparison of assessments of fitness to drive for people with dementia. In: *Neuropsychological rehabilitation* 24 (5), S. 770–783. DOI: 10.1080/09602011.2014.903197.

Wollny, Anja (2008): Demenz. DEGAM - Leitlinie Nr. 12. Düsseldorf: omnikron publishing.

Thank you for your attention!

The pictures were replaced by royalty free pictures from pixabay.com

BEI GRIN MACHT SICH IHR WISSEN BEZAHLT

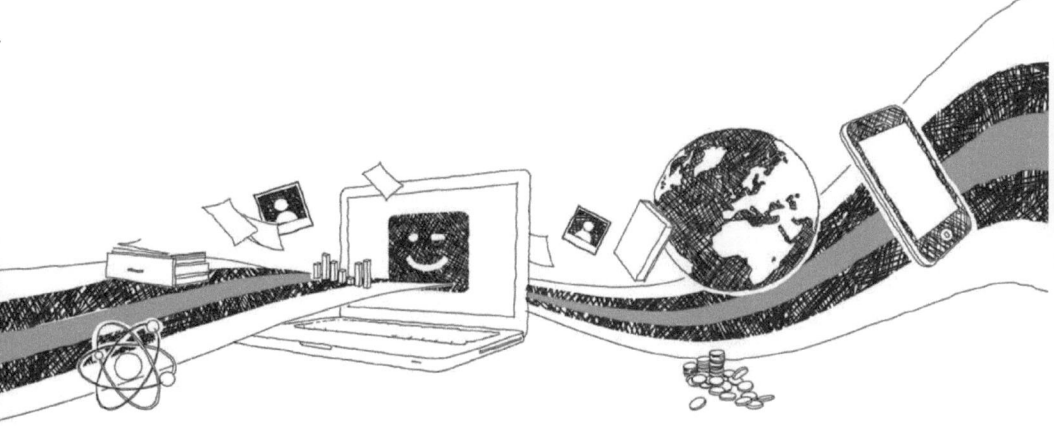

- Wir veröffentlichen Ihre Hausarbeit,
  Bachelor- und Masterarbeit

- Ihr eigenes eBook und Buch -
  weltweit in allen wichtigen Shops

- Verdienen Sie an jedem Verkauf

Jetzt bei www.GRIN.com hochladen und kostenlos publizieren

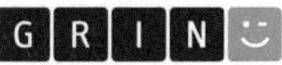